Complete Guide to Herbal Teas

Types of Herbal Teas

Copyright © 2021

DEDICATION

Contents

What Is Herbal Tea? 1

Origins Of Herbal Tea 3

Caffeine Content of Herbal Tea 5

Health Benefits Of Herbal Tea 7

How To Steep Herbal Tea 9

Herbal Tea Recipes 10

What Is Herbal Tea?

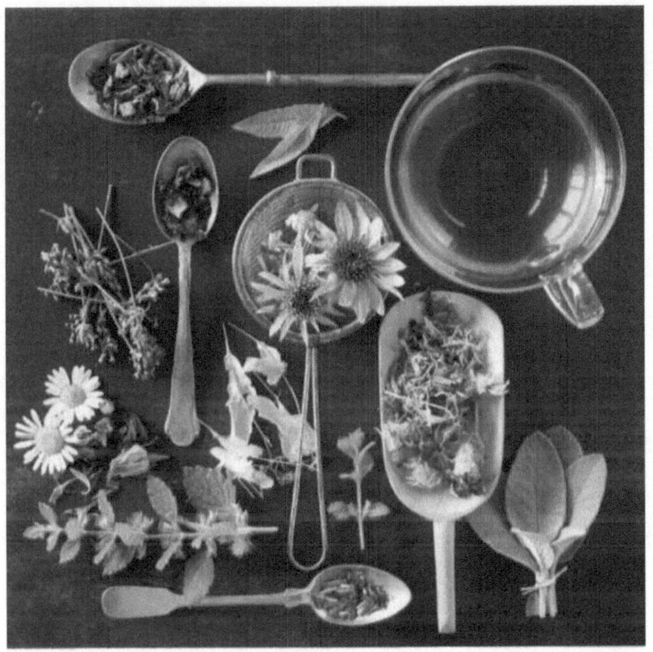

Herbal tea is not technically a true tea, as it does not derive from the Camellia sinensis plant (i.e. the plant that is used to create black, oolong, green, and white teas).

Instead, herbal tea is an infusion or blend of various leaves, fruits, bark, roots, or flowers belonging to almost any edible, non-tea plant. In Europe and other areas of the world, herbal teas are commonly known as tisanes.

Herbal teas have existed for a very long time, but have surged in popularity over the past several decades thanks to their vibrant flavor, as well as their myriad mental, emotional, and physical health benefits. In an increasingly stressful and chaotic world, herbal teas present an opportunity to go back to basics and focus on wellness through a holistic approach.

Because they can be created from almost any combination of natural ingredients, there are a vast number of herbal tea varieties Each with their own flavor qualities and health benefits. Some of the most common herbal teas include:

Chamomile tea

Hibiscus tea

Peppermint tea

Red rooibos tea

Turmeric tea

Spearmint tea

Ginger tea

Yerba maté

Herbal teas are most commonly consumed hot, but they can also be chilled and served over ice, depending on your preferences.

Origins Of Herbal Tea

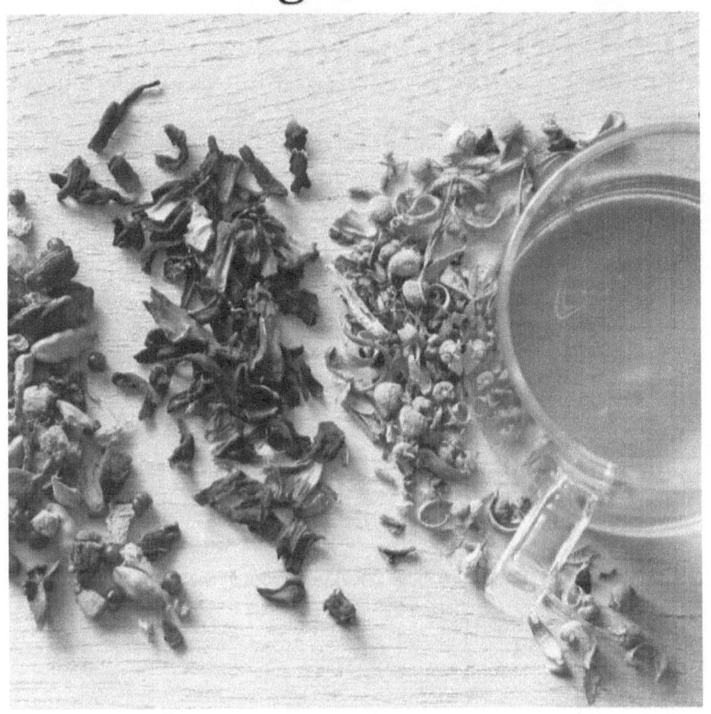

Herbal teas have been around for nearly as long as time. With our ancient ancestors making infusions of the plants, roots, and herbs they saw around them in their native environments. Documentation of herbal teas goes back as far as ancient Egypt and China, where texts have been discovered describing the medicinal benefits of drinking these herbal concoctions.

In the 1st century AD, the legendary Greek physician Dioscorides described more than 600 medicinal plants, many of which could be steeped in water to create healing infusions. Additionally, modern researchers have found dried peppermint leaves in several Egyptian pyramids, which date back to 1,000 BC. Experts believe these were used to aid in digestion.

According to ancient historical records, these herbal blends were used not only for their physical health benefits, but also for their ability to invoke a sense of calm and spiritual awareness. Over time, humans began drinking herbal teas simply for their wonderful taste and aromas.

The practice of using dried herbs, flowers, fruits, barks, and other ingredients for wellness continues today. Many Citizens use herbal teas to support a healthy mind and body.

Caffeine Content of Herbal Tea

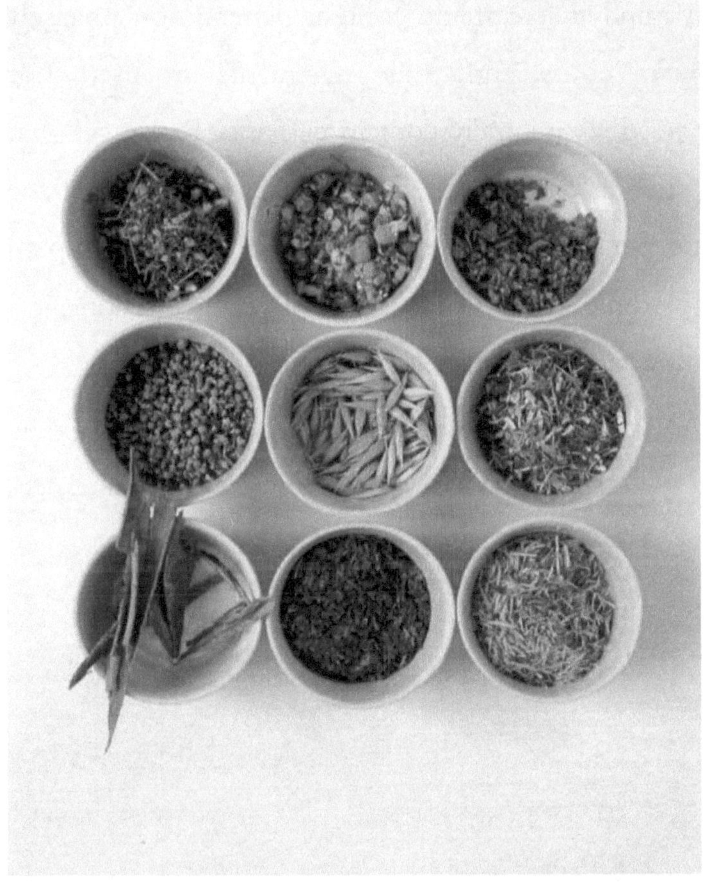

Most varieties of herbal tea — such as chamomile, peppermint, rooibos, and hibiscus — are naturally caffeine-free. For that reason, those who are sensitive to caffeine or who choose to limit their intake often prefer herbal teas over coffee. Additionally, even coffee-lovers may choose to drink tea later in the day, such as before bed, so they can avoid annoying jitters and excess energy while trying to sleep.

However, keep in mind that caffeine content depends on precisely which herbs, flowers, roots, and other ingredients are used. For example, yerba mate does naturally contain caffeine. Beverages that feature this herb, such as the Maté Latte®, contain roughly half the amount of caffeine per cup that is found in a similar-sized cup of coffee. Many people enjoy this gentler burst of energy, making it a popular morning alternative to coffee.

Health Benefits Of Herbal Tea

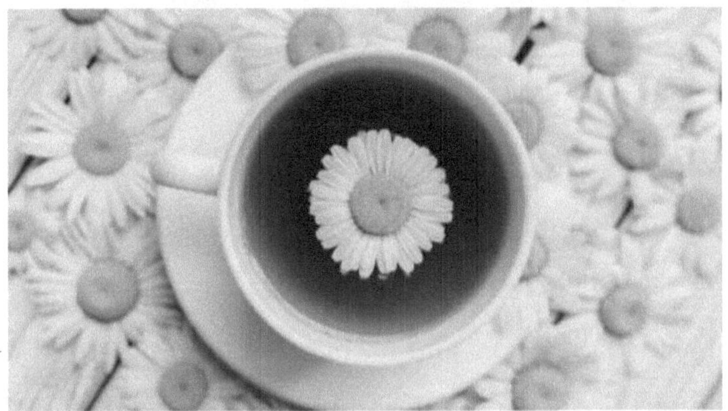

The benefits of herbal teas are as numerous and varied as the herbs themselves. Knowing which benefits you may like to achieve – such as sleeping better, soothing joint pain, or overcoming sluggishness – can help you narrow down the list of options and choose the right herbal blend for your individual needs.

One of the main reasons why herbal tea is so celebrated is because it allows people to reap the health benefits of various herbs, spices and plants through a format that is easy to consume and digest. Most people would find it quite difficult (and not particularly pleasant) to consume healthful ingredients like cinnamon or lavender in their raw form. But by steeping them into a tasty warm beverage, you can easily add these spices and flowers into your diet on a daily basis in a way that is both enjoyable and sustainable.

So, exactly which health benefits do herbal teas deliver? Chamomile tea is known for its calming effect; dandelion tea is known to soothe upset stomachs and aid in digestion; and reishi mushroom tea and red rooibos tea are known for their high concentration of antioxidants.* Ginger, ginseng, turmeric, cinnamon, holy basil, rosehip and ginkgo biloba are examples of other herbal tea varieties, each having their own unique health benefits.*

Some teas may help soothe cold symptoms, while others may help to relieve stress.* In other words, there is an herbal tea to complement every lifestyle, every taste preference, and every wellness goal.

As always, if you have questions about specific herbs it's recommended to consult with your doctor before sipping.

How To Steep Herbal Tea

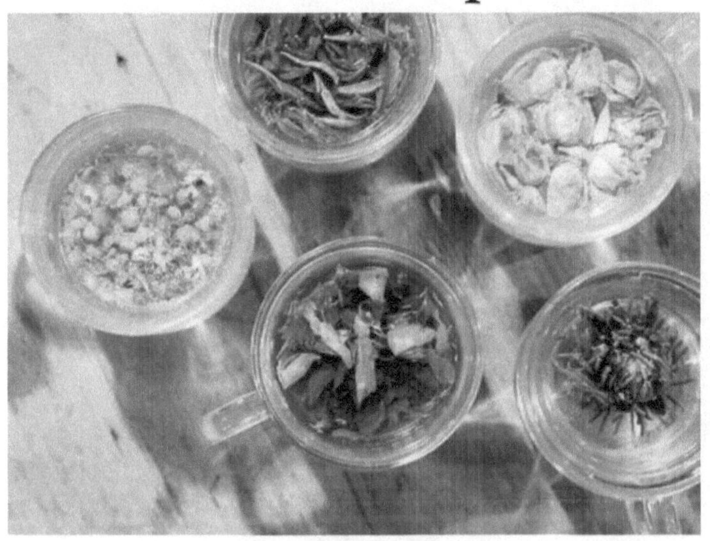

Steeping herbal tea is easy. Simply heat fresh, filtered water to a rolling boil, and set aside about one teaspoon of herbal tea (or one tea bag) per six-ounce cup.

Pour the heated water over the tea, and allow to steep for 5-7 minutes. Then enjoy sip by sip, savoring the flavor and taking note of any mental or physical wellness benefits that you notice. Experiment with steeping times and tea concentrations to find your preferred method.

Herbal Tea Recipes

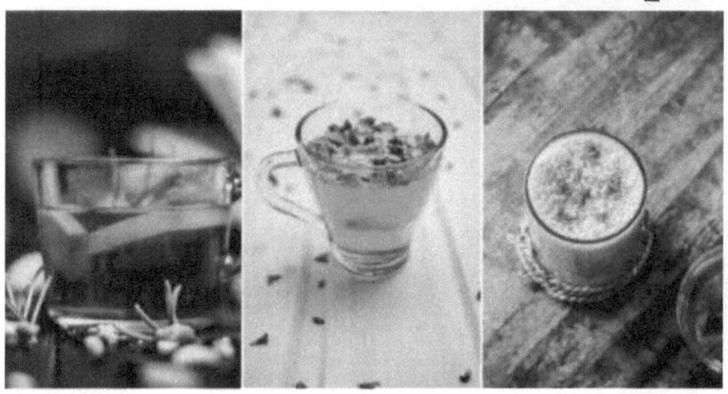

Herbal tea can be used to make a variety of recipes including spritzers, cookies, smoothies, sauces, puddings, and other beverages or desserts. After doing a little research, I found a whole range of different teas with ingredients proven to treat different things, all of which can be made in the comfort of your very own kitchen.

Anti-inflammatory Weight Loss Tea

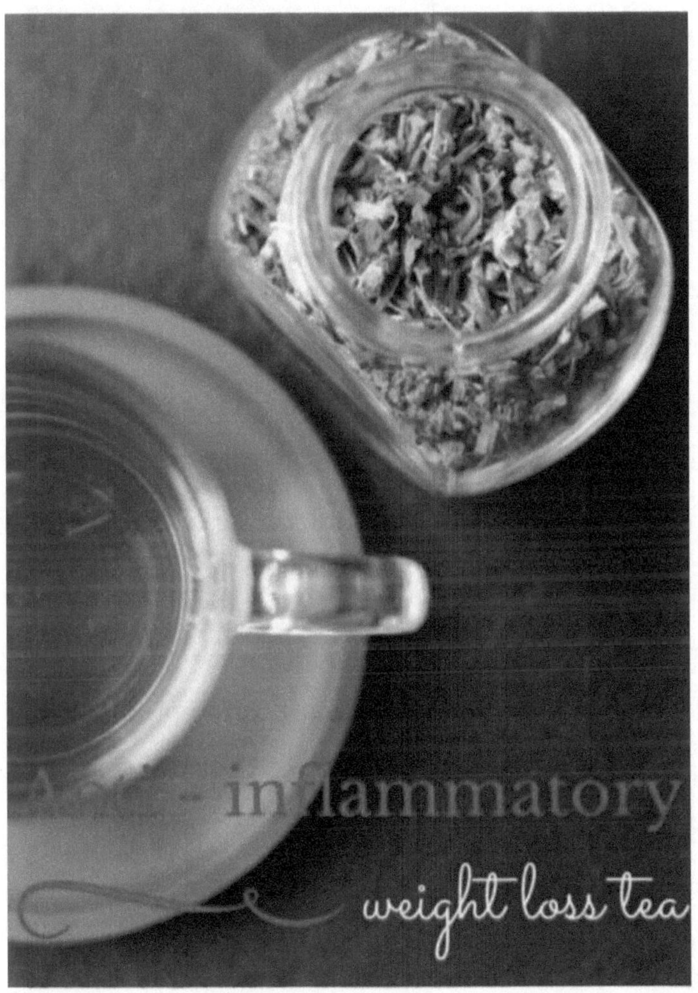

My fingers were swollen for an entire month. I had been reluctantly taking dr prescribed meds but they weren't helping. Then I decided to experiment with some herbs. I came up with this combination and started drinking it religiously.

After 1 week the swelling reduced and unexpectedly my pants were fitting looser around the waist. After 2 weeks of drinking the tea I got up on the scale and to my surprise I had dropped 6 pounds! Keep in mind that because my fingers were swollen so badly I wasn't even going to the gym or doing any exercise, just drinking this tea and eating clean of course.

The diuretic properties of this anti-inflammatory weight loss tea will help to reduce bloating and water weight. I must warn you that it will make you go frequently to the bathroom, that's why I usually have this tea first thing in the morning. If you can get your hands on these herbs I highly recommend this infusion.

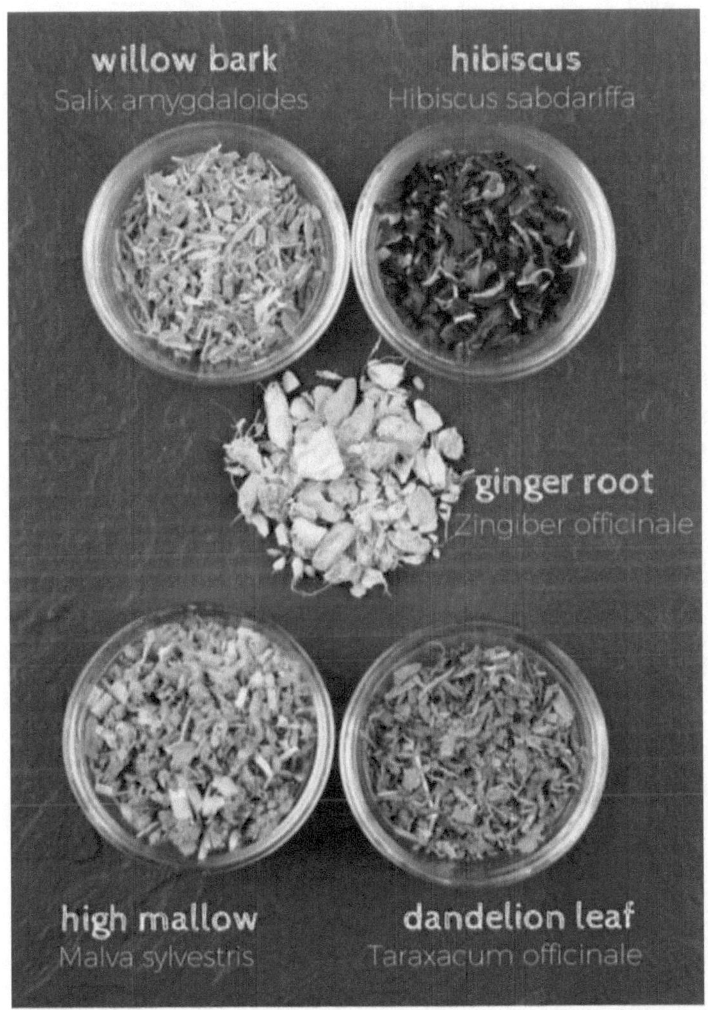

As someone who suffers from occasional joint pain and swelling I can tell you that this anti-inflammatory weight loss tea has been a lifesaver!

Hibiscus (Hibiscus sabdariffa)

Anti-inflammatory and antibacterial properties

Diuretic properties to improve digestion

Promotes weight loss by lowering the absorption of starch and glucose

Relief from cramps and menstrual pain

Ginger root (Zingiber officinale)

Anti-inflammatory

Promotes digestion and stimulates metabolism, which leads to increased calorie burning

Willow bark (Salix amygdaloides)

The active ingredient in willow bark is salicin, which is the same helpful additive in aspirin

Ancient Egyptians used white willow as a folk remedy for inflammation, headaches, menstrual cramps, muscle pain, osteoarthritis, and rheumatoid arthritis. It can also treat the common cold, fever, and assist with weight loss

Dandelion leaf (Taraxacum officinale)

Anti-inflammatory agent for the respiratory tract, the skin, and the gastrointestinal tract.

Diuretic in nature, promotes urination and thereby helps lose "water weight"

High mallow (Malva sylvestris)

Astringent, anti-bacterial and anti-inflammatory properties

Used in traditional herbal medicine for the treatment of gallstones, kidney stones, kidney inflammation, headache, constipation, gastritis, toothaches and insomnia.

INGREDIENTS

Equal amounts of

Dried hibiscus flowers

Dried ginger root

Organic dried willow bark

Organic dried dandelion leaf

High Mallow (Malva sylvestris)

INSTRUCTIONS

Combine all herbs in a tight closing jar and store in a cool dark place.

For each serving of tea, steep 1 tablespoon of the mixture together with 1 cup hot water for 3 to 5 minutes.

Energy Herbal Tea

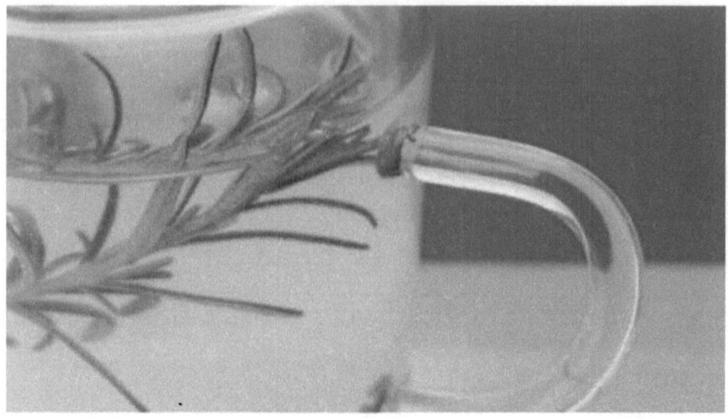

This recipe for Energy Herbal Tea looks delicious, with both sweet and herbal aspects to it.

<u>INGREDIENTS</u>

1/2 teaspoon loose green tea leaves

1 teaspoon rosemary

1/8 teaspoon nutmeg

Honey (optional)

8 ounces water

<u>INSTRUCTIONS</u>

Add to infuser and steep for 5-7 minutes.

Sweeten with honey if desired.

Chamomile and Turmeric Evening Tea

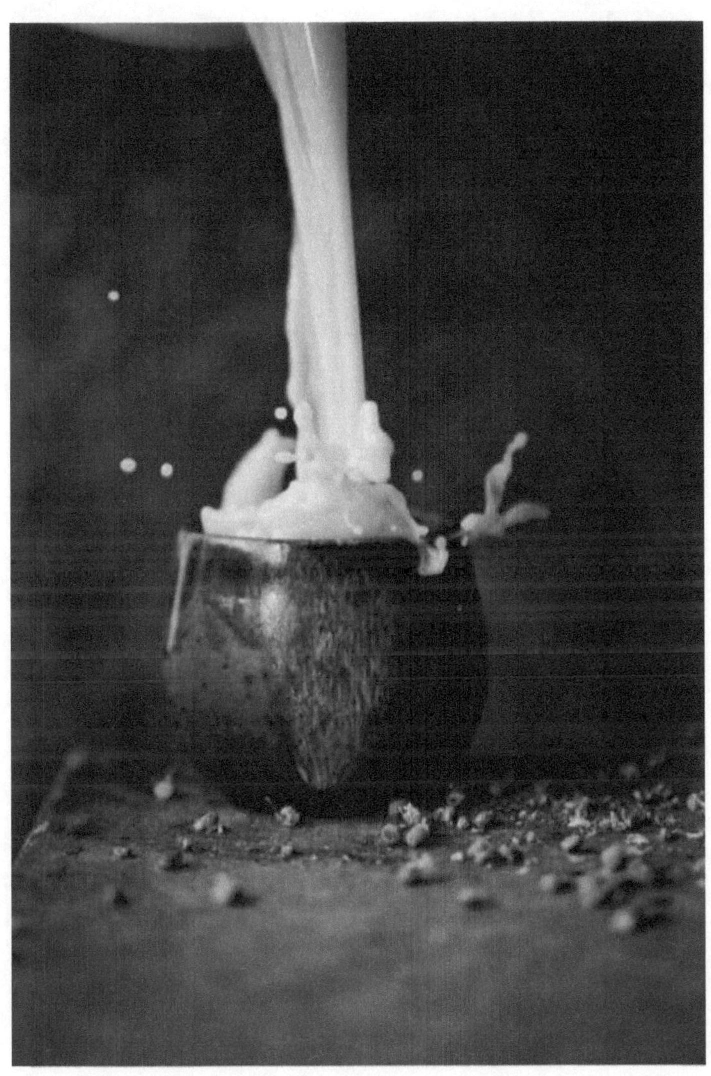

We made this tea part of our evening routine while we were driving around the chillier south island of New Zealand. It was the perfect way to end the day after having driven for hours, taken mountain hikes and played on the windy sand beaches. Sitting on wobbly plastic chairs next to the car, watching the sunset and drinking this warm and soothing evening tea before going to bed. Oh happy memories!

Warm chamomile tea with honey is indeed a good sleep-aid. Chamomile is calming and honey is anti-bacterial. We kept a huge jar New Zealand Manuka with us in the van and it felt like such a luxury. Active Manuka honey is known for its medicinal properties. If you can't find it or afford it, choose another unheated quality honey. Coconut oil is a true super food with a long list of health benefits, add it to your daily routine and always choose a cold pressed quality oil. It gives tea a round and rich consistency and leaves you more satisfied. It can however feel a little oily and unusual if you are not used to it, so I recommend starting with a little less. Turmeric, ginger and cinnamon add great flavour as well as immune-boosting and anti-inflammatory properties. Try adding a little black pepper, the black pepper helps to enhance the bioavailability of curcumin in turmeric by a thousand times.

<u>INGREDIENTS</u>

2 cups drinking water

2 tbsp dried chamomile in a tea bag or 2 chamomile tea sachets (organic if possible)

1-3 tsp cold-pressed coconut oil

1 1/2 cup unsweetened plant milk of choice

1/2 tsp ground turmeric

1/4 tsp ground ginger

1/4 tsp ground cinnamon

(a pinch of black pepper, optional)

1 tbsp raw honey (Manuka honey if possible) or more to taste

<u>INSTRUCTIONS</u>

Bring water to a boil in a sauce pan. Turn off the heat, then add chamomile and let steep for 3-5 minutes. Discard the chamomile. Now stir in milk, coconut oil, turmeric, ginger, cinnamon, (black pepper) and honey. Taste and add more honey, coconut oil or spices if you prefer. Re-heat on low heat if needed.

Banana Tea

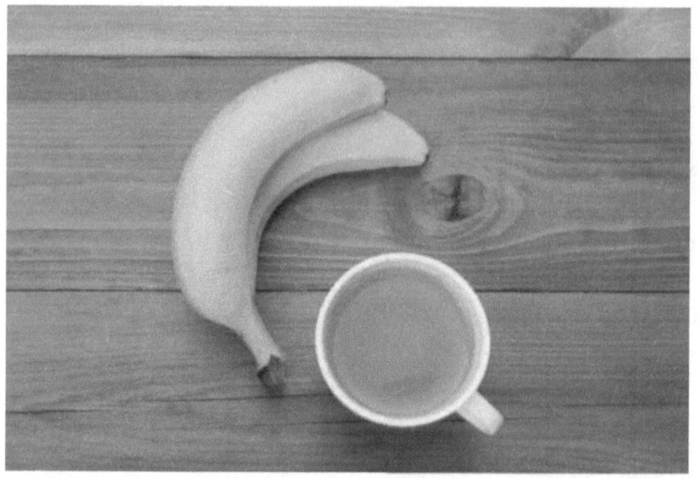

Did you know bananas are a sleeping pill in a peel? If you find yourself waking up in the middle of the night, try this banana-infused tea as a bedtime snack. Studies have shown that magnesium can be helpful in preventing you from pulling yourself out of sleep, and the potassium and magnesium help your blood vessels and muscles relax.

INGREDIENTS

1 raw banana

1 small pot of water

sprinkle of cinnamon (optional)

INSTRUCTIONS

Boil water. Cut off both ends of banana and place in water. Boil for about 10 minutes.

Pour water through colander and into mug. Drink one hour before bed.

If you're feeling adventurous, you can also eat the banana and its peel an hour before bed. For an extra flavor kick, sprinkle with cinnamon!

Herbal Chai Tea

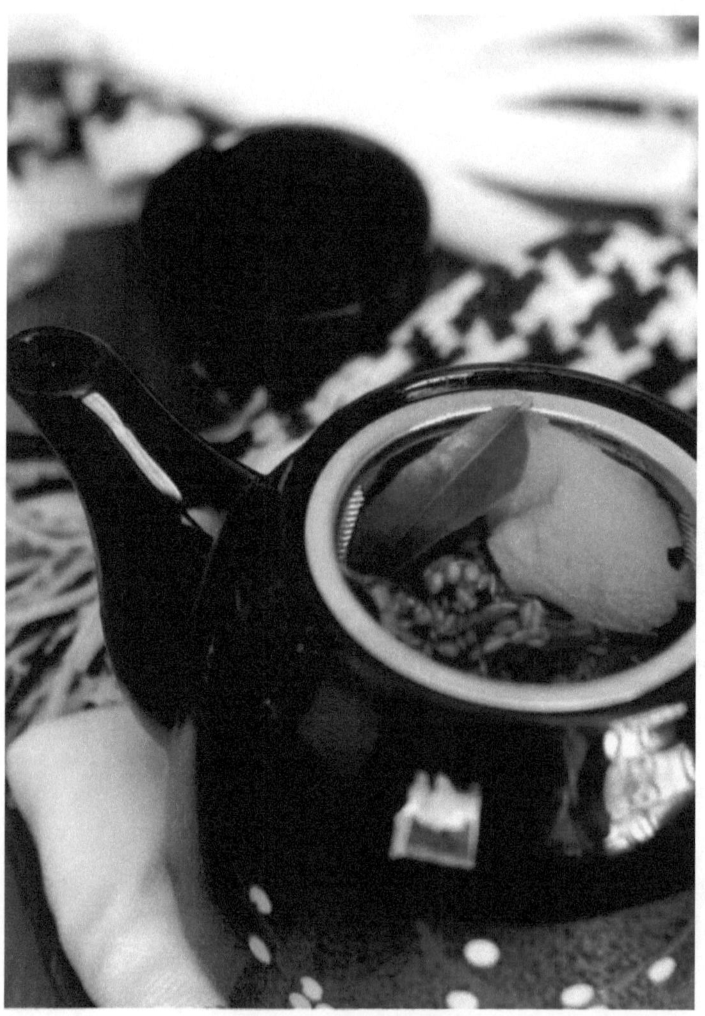

Herbal chai tea is the perfect home remedy to soothe your aching throats, and the congestion in your nose and chest. With the cold and flu season at its peak, it is a good idea to keep this tea ready and handy but be warned, you must double your batch. The non-sick people at home will be drinking the winter away with this insanely-feel good herbal chai tea!

<u>INGREDIENTS</u>

1/4 cup crudely sliced and crushed ginger

15-20 curry leaves (available at Asian Stores)

1 tbsp coriander seeds (Sabut Dhaniya)

1 tbsp cumin seeds (Jeera)

1 tsp celery seeds (ajwain)

A pinch of turmeric

1/2 tsp whole black pepper (Kaali Mirch)

1/4 tsp cloves

5-6 cups of water

<u>INSTRUCTIONS</u>

Add all the ingredients in a pot and let the water reach a boil.

Set the heat on medium, cover & cook until the water level reduces to about 2/3rd.

Pour into a teapot and serve

This can be served two ways:

• with a tsp of honey and a dollop of milk

• with a pinch of salt and a dash of lemon juice

<u>MY TAKE</u>

If you happen to have holy basil / Tulsi at home, it makes a great addition both in terms of medicinal value and flavor to the tea.

Apple Fig Herbal Tea

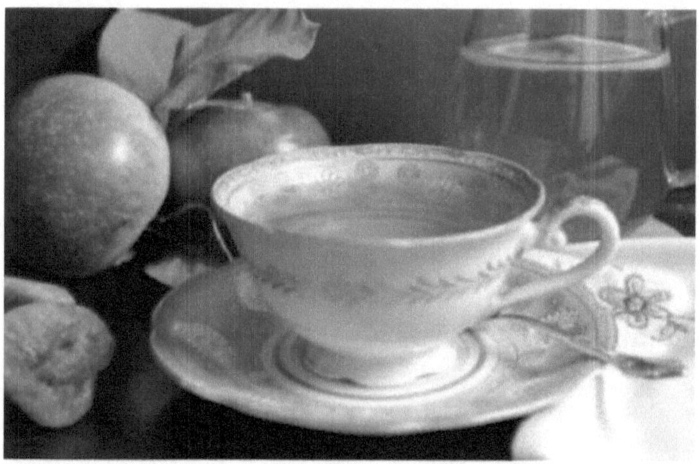

A tradition can usually be defined as a behavior or a belief that is passed down from generation to generation. Traditions are usually predictable and they have the power to create a sense of unity. Often, traditions are associated with some of the best memories of our lives and as you are probably aware, food and tradition go hand in hand. I would like to share with you a hot beverage which is traditional in my family. I have called it Apple Fig Herbal Tea.

Hope you get a chance to try this recipe for an apple fig herbal tea. It just might become a tradition in your family.

<u>INGREDIENTS</u>

8 cups water

3-4 apples washed and quartered

6-8 dried figs

Lemon wedge optional

Honey optional

Cinnamon stick optional

<u>INSTRUCTIONS</u>

Place water, apples and dried figs in a large pot.

Bring to boil.

Reduce heat and simmer for 1-1 1/2 hours.

Strain and serve.

Adjust to taste with lemon wedge, honey and/or cinnamon.

<u>NOTES</u>

I usually make a big batch and refrigerate any leftovers. The longer the tea simmers, the sweeter the taste.

Herbal Tea for Allergies

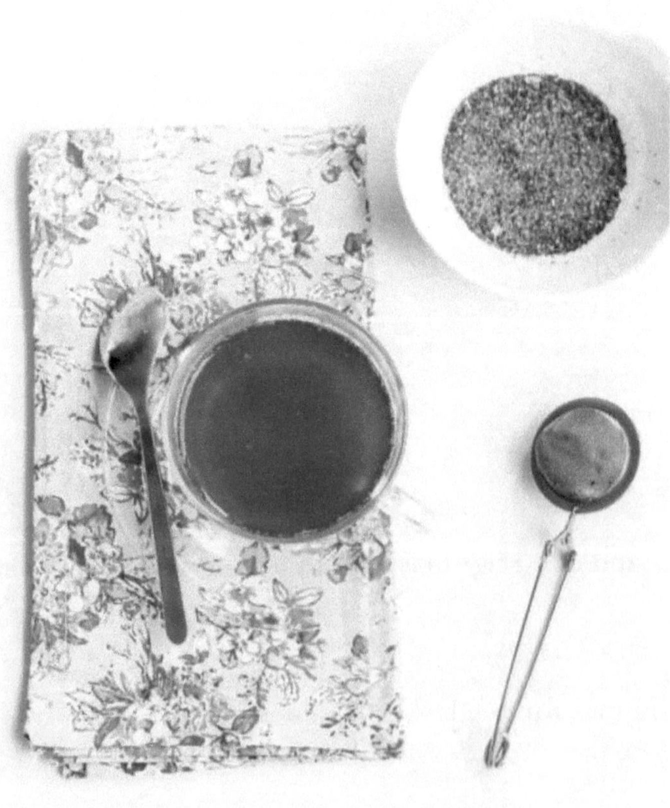

First, let's talk about the different components and what they do.

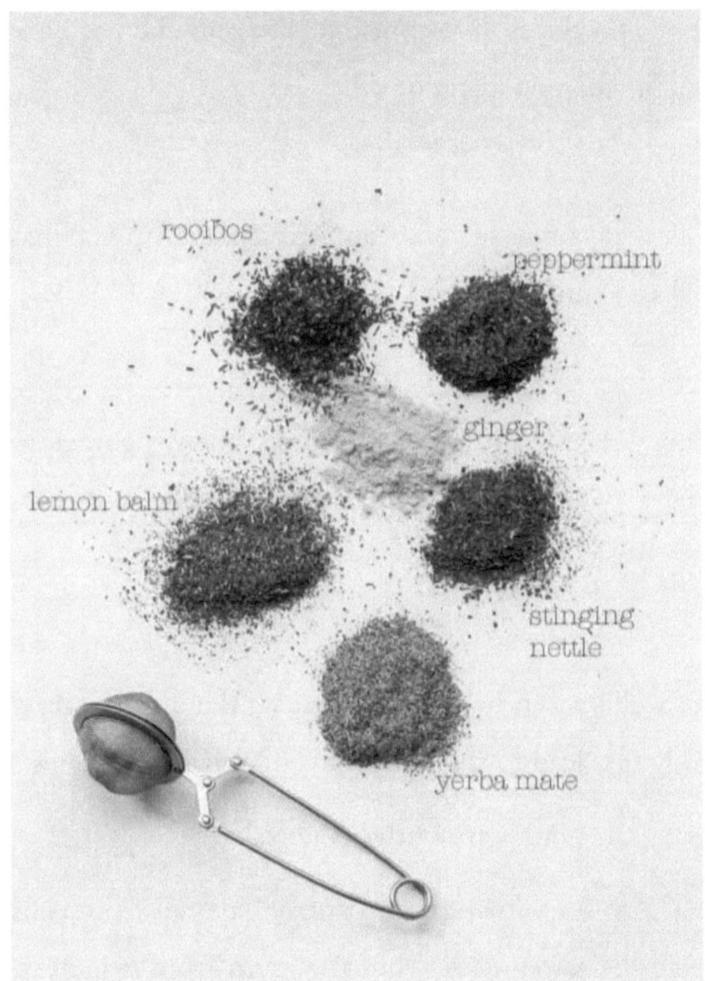

Rooibos

Rooibos, also called Red Bush Tea, comes from South Africa. It is naturally caffeine-free and contains two bioflavonoids called rutin and quercetin. Both of these compounds block the release of histamine, the chemical our body produces in response to allergens and has been shown to have benefits for skin irritations.

Peppermint

Peppermint acts as a decongestant, an anti-inflammatory, and has known antibacterial and antiviral effects

Dried ginger

Ginger has so many amazing healing properties! When it comes to allergies and colds, it works as a natural antihistamine and anti-inflammatory

Stinging Nettle

Nettles have a very well known beneficial effect on the inflammatory pathways in the body that lead to the symptoms of seasonal allergies.

Drinking tea or eating the nettles are both beneficial.

You might have less than fond memories of stinging nettles from your childhood. These are the same nettles, but they turn from irritant to healer when boiled into tea. Boiling fresh nettles will remove the stinging properties, while taking them in capsule, fresh, or dried form can help relieve itchy, watery eyes, sneezing, and runny nose.

Yerba mate

Yerba Mate is very popular in South America. It contains natural caffeine and acts as an anti-inflammatory in response to allergens. This can help to open up respiratory passages and increase oxygen.

Lemon balm

Lemon balm belongs to the mint family but has a lemony scent, hence, its name. It's calming, and it can help with headaches, the common cold, and other respiratory issues. In animal models, it has been shown to relieve some of the swelling of the tissues that takes place in inflammatory processes, and that could be beneficial in allergies.

Honey & Lemon

Contrary to popular belief, honey doesn't actually help combat allergies, but it can soothe an itchy throat. In a study with subjects suffering from the four main allergy symptoms, nasal congestion, nasal itchiness, runny nose, and sneezing, honey helped their antihistamine work much better to improve all of them. It seems it can also inhibit the action of the cells causing those symptoms in this study on honey-bee collected pollen's effects on mast cells.

I like to use local raw honey, but the regular kind will help coat a sore throat, too. The lemon acts as a detoxifier and source of vitamin C to boost immunity. You can add one or both to your herbal tea for allergies.

Here are some simple herbal tea infusions you can make to help you get through spring allergy season. They can be taken hot or turned into an iced tea.

<u>EQUIPMENT</u>

Glass jar with lid or other airtight container

Tea kettle

<u>INGREDIENTS</u>

All-Purpose Allergy Blend

1 part rooibos

1 part peppermint tea

1 part nettle tea

1 part yerba mate

1 part lemon balm tea

Antihistamine Tea

1 bag stinging nettle tea

1 bag peppermint tea

1/2 teaspoon ground ginger you can use grated fresh ginger, too

<u>INSTRUCTIONS</u>

Mix ingredients together and store in an airtight container.

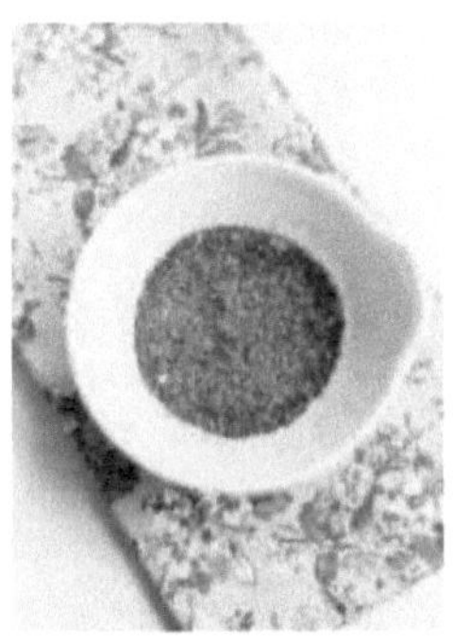

Use about 1 heaping teaspoon per 8 ounces hot water.

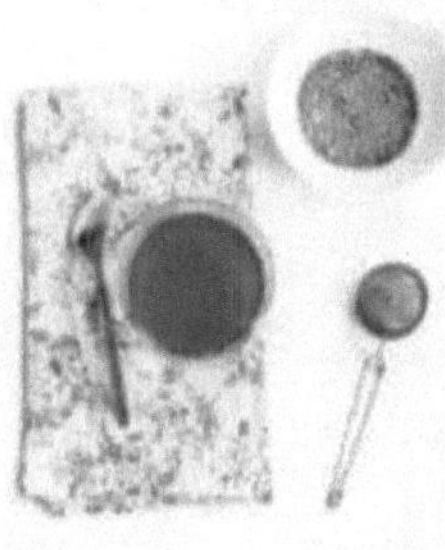

Let steep for about 5 minutes, then add honey or lemon, if desired.

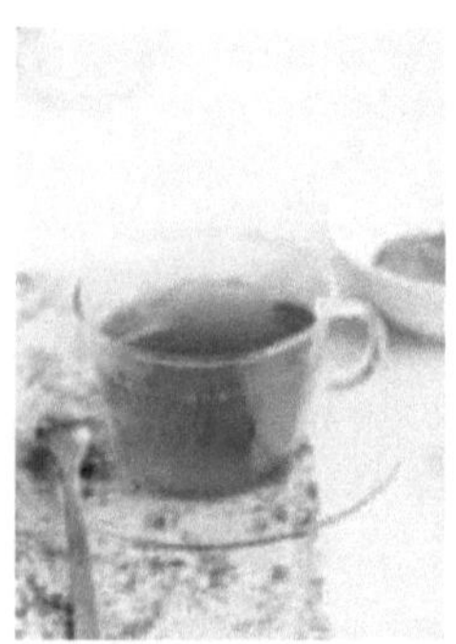

<u>NOTES</u>

Make sure water doesn't exceed 212°F, which is the boiling point at sea level, otherwise it can lessen the effectiveness of the tea.

Licorice Tea

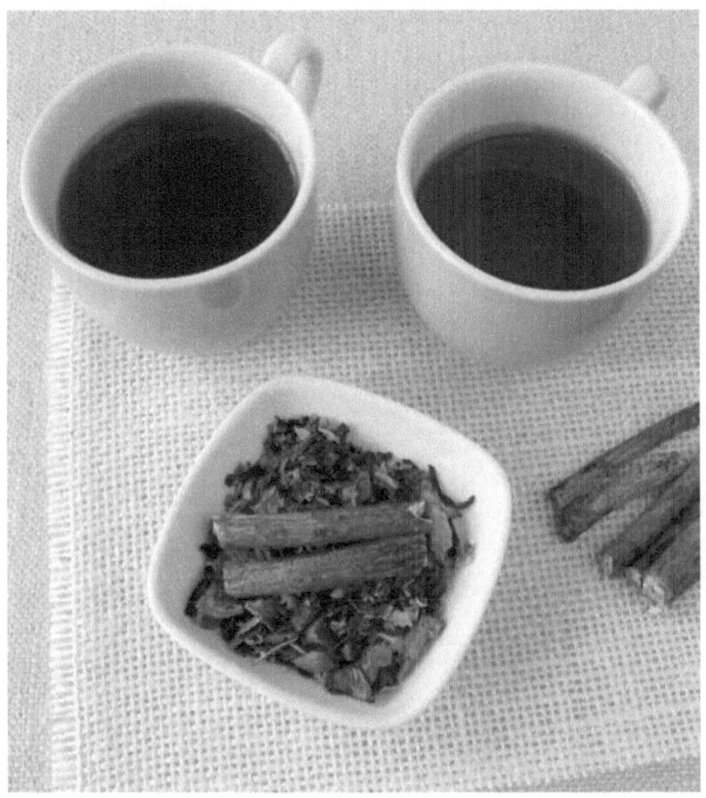

Licorice root tea is made from the root of the medicinal herb licorice (also known as liquorice). It is the most used herb in Chinese medicine and has been used in Europe since prehistoric times. It has been used for centuries to flavor foods, to sweeten drinks, to flavor tobacco, as a foaming agent in beers, and to harmonize contrasting herbs.

Where Does Licorice Root Come From…

The Glycyrrhiza glabra plant (licorice) is a perennial that is native to southern Europe and Asia. The root is harvested and often boiled. In the boiling process, the sweetener glycyrrhizin is removed to form licorice extract which is significantly sweeter than sugar.

Benefits of Licorice Root…

Settles stomach problems – licorice root will help relieve stomach pain, treat ulcer and heartburn, and will jump-start the digestive tract in case of constipation.

Relieve stress and fatigue – licorice can help regulate cortisol which is the stress hormone. As a result, it gives our adrenal glands a break and prevents adrenal fatigue.

Supports a healthy respiratory system – licorice root is anti-inflammatory and will help loosen mucus in the lungs and clear clogged nasal passages. it is very effective in treating cough.

Relieve muscle pain – licorice is antispasmodic and will help relieve cramping in the muscles.

Strengthen the immune system – licorice is both antibacterial and antiviral. It will support and strengthen your immune system making your body stronger against colds and the flu. Licorice is also emerging as a potential treatment and prevention for diseases like hepatitis C,

HIV, and influenza.

Treats tooth decay and prevents cavities – chemical compounds in licorice root help prevent bacteria in oral cavities that cause the formation of plaque and acid which leads to tooth decay. Chewing on licorice root will not only help you keep your teeth healthy but also keep your breath fresh and remove bad odors.

Improves hair and skin health – licorice root contains elements like choline, phytoestrogens, potassium, phosphorus, amines, essential oils, protein, vitamin B, and flavonoids. Those will promote a healthy scalp, hair, and skin. Licorice root is effective in treating dandruff, preventing hair loss, repairing skin damage, and curing eczema and skin rashes.

Reduces PMS, hot flashes, and treats yeast infection – due to its anti-inflammatory and antispasmodic properties licorice can help with PMS. Licorice can help regulate hormones and help with menopause issues like hot flashes and mood swings. Licorice root can also fight and cure yeast infection.

Helps with weight loss and good for diabetics – licorice extract is a natural sweetener that is even sweeter than sugar. If you are diabetic, consider using it to replace sugar in food and drinks. Studies suggest that regular drinking of licorice tea can significantly help reduce body fat mass due to the stomach acid controlling properties of licorice.

Support mental health – licorice contains a compound known as carbenoxolone. This compound inhibits an enzyme that regulates stress hormones in the brain that has been associated with mental decline.

How to Prepare Licorice Root…

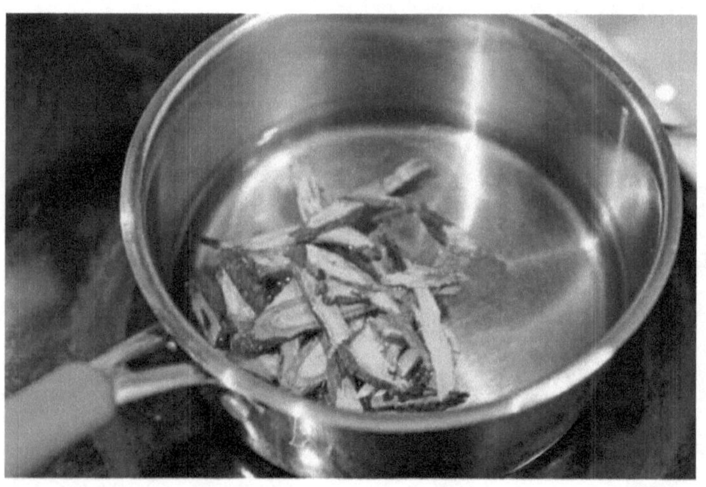

To a pot, add 0.5 oz (=one tablespoon) licorice root for every one cup of water. If you buy the licorice root slices as I use here, it's easier to weight it since it doesn't exactly fit in a teaspoon. If you buy the chopped root, it's easier to add it by the tablespoons.

If you are making the tea to treat a sore throat or a cough, also add a stick of cinnamon and a couple of slices of ginger. There is no need to add any sweetener! Licorice root is very sweet.

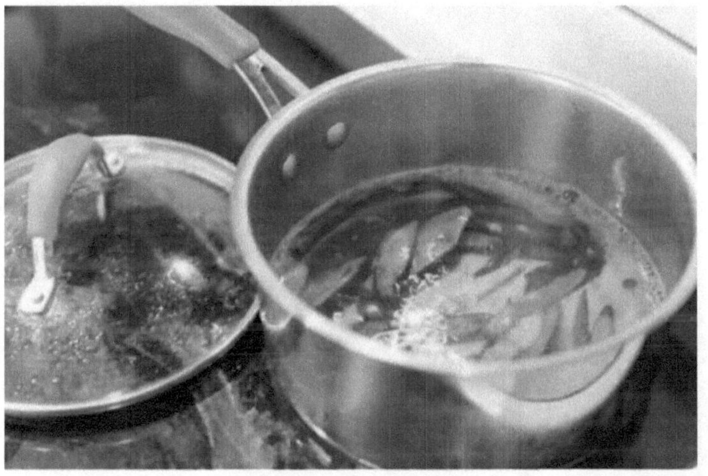

Bring to a boil, then lower the temperature and let it simmer for 10 minutes. Turn the heat off and let the tea rest for 5 minutes.

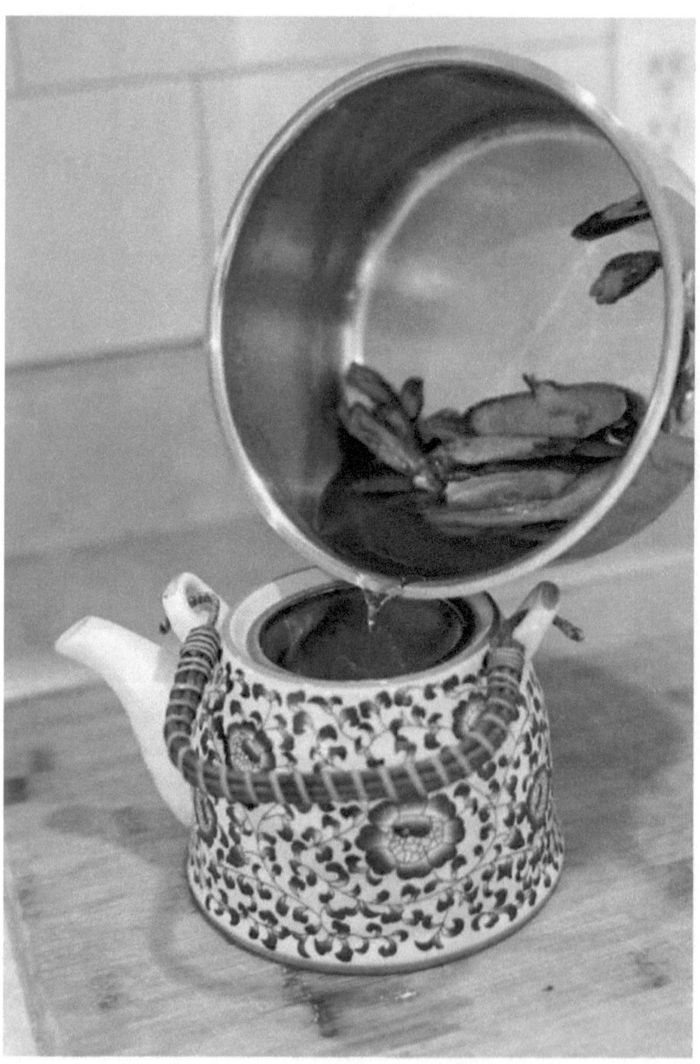

Next, pour your tea through a strainer into a teapot or straight into a cup and enjoy!

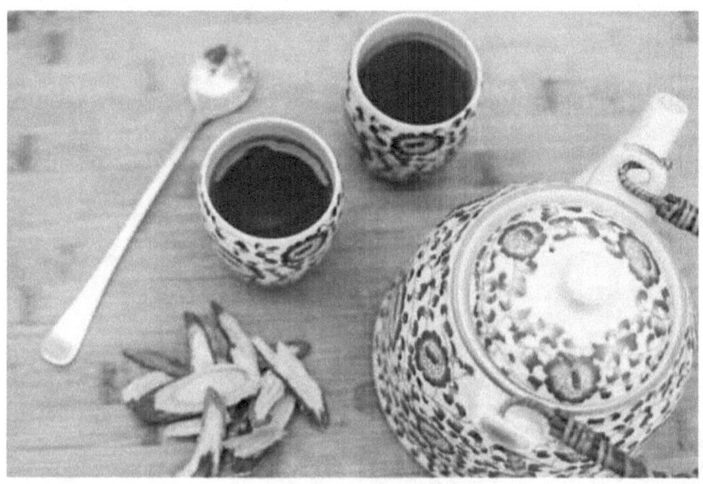

Precautions…

It is advised that young children (under 50lb), pregnant women, and nursing women do not use licorice in any form. Licorice might increase the risk of miscarriage some say, but there is no research to back this up.

Kids that weight more than 50lb can drink 1/3 cup of licorice tea to relieve sore throat and cough up to three times a day for a couple of days.

There are no specific instructions for adults. Just don't overdo it because too much glycyrrhizin can cause serious side effects like headaches, fatigue, and high blood pressure.

If used in moderation regularly, licorice tea can play a big role in keeping your body healthy and strong. We increase the amount we drink right away if we feel that we are getting sick or if someone wakes up with a sore throat (up to three cups a day). Then, once we feel better again, we go back to two or three cups a week.

Honey, Lemon and Ginger Tea

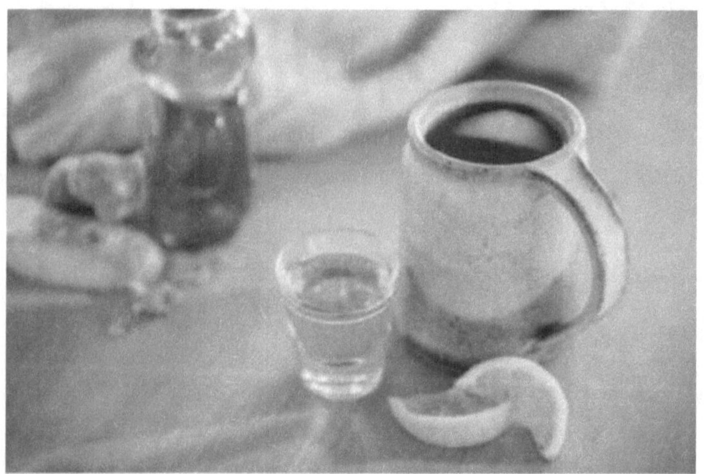

Feeling achy? Stuffy? Sore throat? This patented Honey Lemon Ginger Tea will help. No joke. Well, joke about the patent, but no joke about it helping you feel a bit better if you have a cold or the flu.

The heat and the ginger will warm you right up, the steam—aided by the bright lemon and the potent ginger—will help clear those sinuses, and the ginger and the honey will work to sooth that scratchy throat. If you're feeling old-school, go ahead and add a shot of whiskey to the mix (especially if you're drinking it right before going to bed) for a sort of medicinal hot toddy.

If you're really suffering, try making a triple batch and keep it in a thermos to sip, or reheat it as needed. Want a thoughtful-person-of-the-year award? Make a batch for someone in your house who's suffering.

INGREDIENTS

1-inch fresh ginger root (no need to peel it)

1 cup water (boiling)

1 tablespoon lemon juice (freshly squeezed)

1 tablespoon honey (raw, unpasteurized)

Optional: 1 shot whiskey

INSTRUCTIONS

Gather the ingredients.

Grate the ginger into a teapot, medium bowl or large measuring cup. In most culinary uses, you want to peel ginger, but there really is no reason to do so here, and it will just take time and effort better spent lying down and resting when you're not well. But you do need to grate it (if you're in a really bad way, you can just slice it, but know you won't get nearly as much of a ginger kick that way and you may regret your laziness). Best case scenario: Grate the ginger on a microplane zester. Next best situation: Grate the ginger on the fine holes of a four-sided grater (or similar). What also works: mince the ginger with a sharp knife. Truly fresh, young ginger will be quite tender, with few fibers getting in your way. Older ginger, however, will have a fair amount of fiber running through it. Go ahead and put it all on the pot—you're going to strain it out anyway.

Pour 1 cup boiling water over the ginger and let it steep for 3 minutes.

Meanwhile, put the lemon juice and the honey in a large mug.

Strain the ginger tea into the mug.

Stir to dissolve the honey, taste, and add more honey or lemon juice if you like.

Serve hot.

Weight-Loss Green Tea

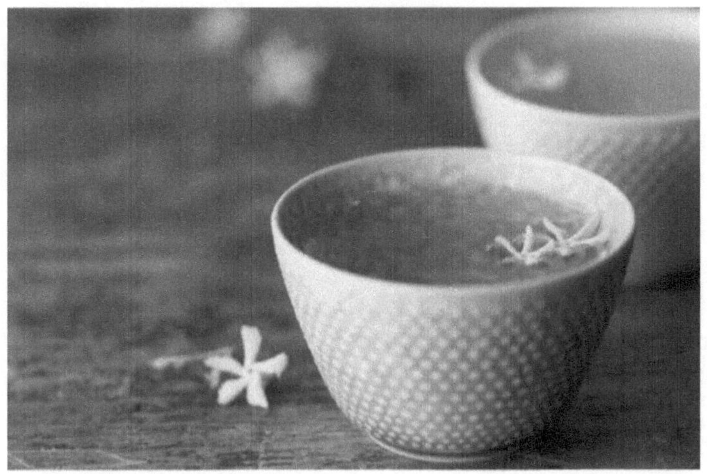

You may be considering adding green tea to your diet to improve your health, lose weight or manage a specific medical condition. While green tea may aid weight loss efforts, it is not a magic bullet, and it needs to be combined with other lifestyle changes.

Green Tea Benefits

All types of tea come from the Camellia sinensis plant, but different types of tea undergo various levels of processing. Because making green tea only involves steaming the leaves, it is the least processed of all the teas, which makes it high in antioxidants.

While much more research is needed, consuming green tea may help to lower the risk of certain types of cancer, improve alertness, improve cholesterol levels, lower the risk of heart disease and aid weight loss, says the National Center for Complementary and Alternative Medicine. Green tea is considered generally safe; however, you should always speak to your physician about the safety of any herbal product before using it.

Green Tea and Belly Fat

While much more research is needed, certain chemicals in green tea called polyphenols and, more specifically, the catechins, may boost metabolism and help burn fat. The best results seem to occur in those who are overweight or moderately obese and drink a combination of green tea and caffeine.

A general recommendation is to consume 2 to 3 cups of green tea per day or a total of 240 to 320 milligrams of polyphenols. If you are sensitive to caffeine, however, this may be too much to consume each day.

Green Tea Extracts

Green tea can also be taken in supplement form. While green tea is considered generally safe, there is not enough evidence to fully support claims that it aids weight loss, reports the Mayo Clinic. However, the active chemicals in green tea are thought to not only improve calorie and fat metabolism, but they may also help to suppress your appetite.

Even if green tea or green tea extracts do support weight loss, you must still watch your calorie intake and get regular exercise to fully control your weight.

Lemon and Weight Loss

Adding lemon to your green tea may help to improve the taste if you so desire. In addition, lemon may also act as a natural appetite suppressant.

The bottom line in weight loss, however, is that you must take in fewer calories than you burn. Those who are successful at long-term weight loss combine watching what they eat with regular moderate-level exercise on most days of the week.

While adding green tea with lemon into your diet plan may help, green tea can interact with other medications you're taking, so it should only be used under medical supervision.

<u>INGREDIENTS</u>

2 mugs drinking water

Fennel seeds (2 tbsp)

Green tea bag (any) i had Moroccan mint flavoured green tea

Ginger (2 small pieces)

Honey (optional)

<u>INSTRUCTIONS</u>

In a pot boil all the ingredients. When colour changes. Turn off the flame. And pour in mug. Serve hot.

Cinnamon Sleep Tonic

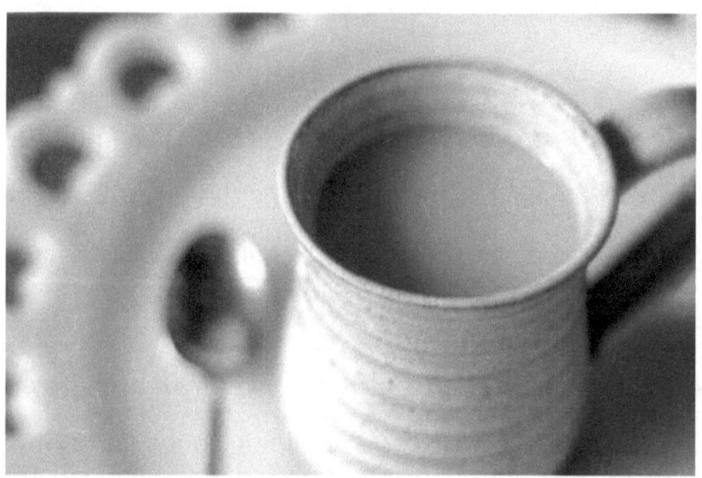

<u>INGREDIENTS</u>

– 3 cinnamon sticks

– 1 tablespoon all-spice berries

– 1 tablespoon cloves

– 1/2 teaspoon peppercorns (optional)

– 15 bay leaves

– 2" piece of fresh ginger, cut into large pieces

– 10 cups filtered water

<u>INSTRUCTIONS</u>

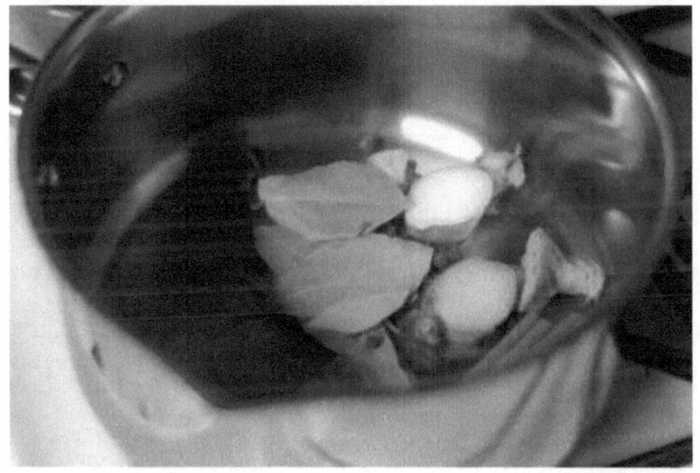

Step One: Combine all the ingredients together in a large saucepan. Bring to a boil, reduce heat, and allow them to steep for 2-3 hours.

Step Two: Drink. Either plain or with a dollop of fresh cream, coconut oil, butter, or honey.

Green Tea

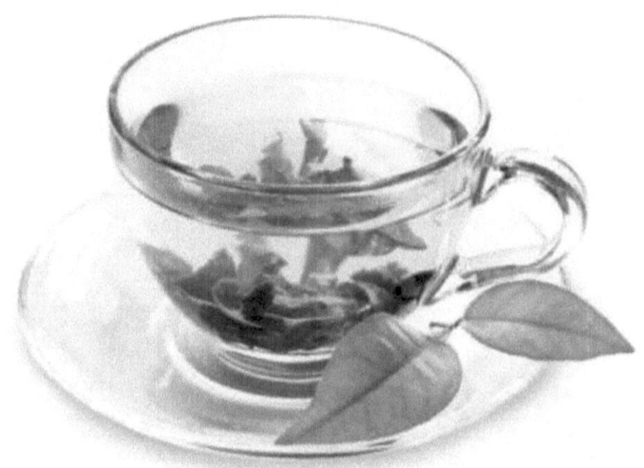

How To Prepare Green Tea With Leaves

Green tea preparation is different than that of black tea that we make at home. You need to follow some simple steps. While making green tea, do keep in mind that if the tea leaves are steeped in water that's over 90°C, the tea will become bitter. So, steep it in water that's not too hot. Here are the steps for green tea brewing with leaves.

<u>INGREDIENTS</u>

Green tea leaves – the basic quantity would be 1 teaspoon for 1 cup of green tea. You may also use green tea pearls.

A tea strainer. Wash and dry it – this step is necessary if you use this strainer to make regular black tea.

A cup

A stainless steel pot

1 cup of water

<u>INSTRUCTIONS</u>

Step 1

Take one teaspoon of green tea leaves. If you want to make more than a cup of green tea, take 1 teaspoon of green tea leaves for each cup. So, take 4 teaspoons of green tea leaves for 4 cups of green tea.

Step 2

Now, take the tea leaves in a strainer/sieve and keep aside.

Step 3

Now, take a stainless steel pot/pan and boil the water. If you want to use a glass teapot instead, go ahead. The ideal temperature for green tea is 80°C to 85°C, so keep an eye on the water to make sure it's not boiling. If it starts boiling anyway, just switch off the gas/heat and let it cool for a bit (say, for 30-45 seconds).

Step 4

Now, place the sieve/ strainer over the cup or mug.

Step 5

Next, pour the hot water into the cup and let the tea steep for 3 minutes. This is the step where we need to be very careful. Not everyone likes their tea strong, so, to check whether the tea is just right, keep a spoon handy and drink a spoonful of tea every 30-45 seconds to find out if the flavor is right for you.

Step 6

Now, take out the sieve and keep it aside. If you want, you may add 1 teaspoon honey.

Step 7

Stir the honey in and let the drink cool for a few seconds. Enjoy your cup of green tea.

How To Make Green Tea With Tea Bags

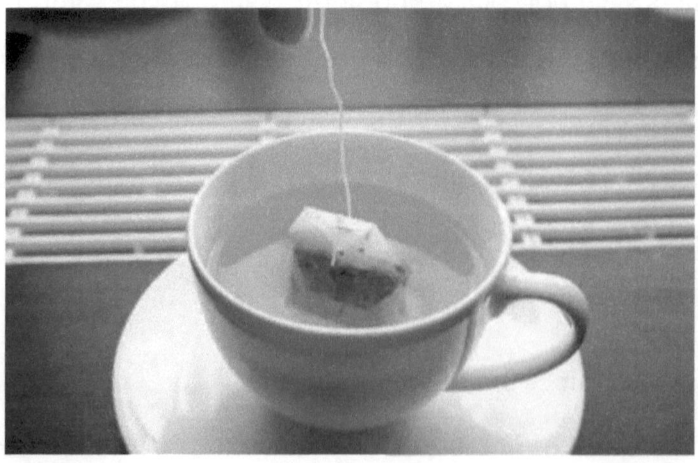

Green tea bags are, well, convenient for many people. They are portable and can be made into a hot cuppa quickly – all you need is a cup of hot water. So, here's how you can prepare a cup of green tea with a green tea bag. If you are using tea bags, make sure they are made from an unbleached material. Most tea bags are bleached to make them white, and you definitely don't want any bleach contaminating your antioxidant-rich drink!

<u>INGREDIENTS</u>

1 good quality green tea bag

1 cup of hot water

1 stainless steel/clay cup

A lid to cover the cup

A stainless steel pot

<u>INSTRUCTIONS</u>

Step 1

Heat the water in a stainless steel pot. Make sure it doesn't come to a boiling point, which is 100 degrees C. The temperature of the water should be around 80-85 degrees C.

Step 2

Put the green tea bag into the clay or stainless steel cup.

Step 3

Pour the hot water into the cup and cover it with a small lid. Let it steep for 3 minutes.

Step 4

After 3 minutes is over, remove the lid and remove the tea bag.

Step 5

Stir with a spoon and take a rejuvenating sip!

How To Brew Green Tea With Powder

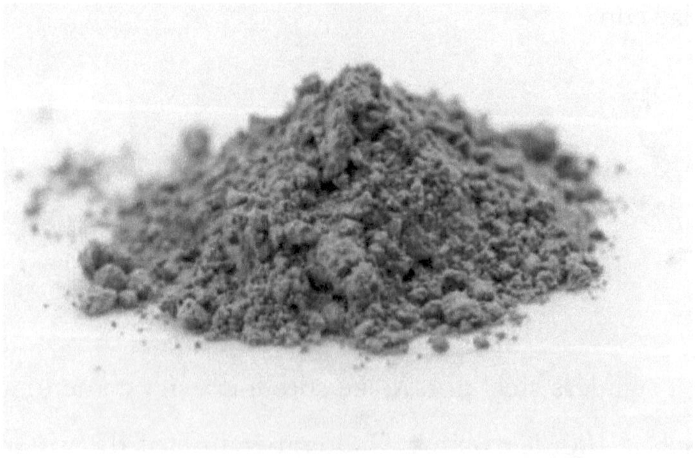

You may also prepare green tea using green tea powder, which is available readily in the market. Here's the best way to make green tea using green tea powder.

<u>INGREDIENTS</u>

Green tea powder – 1 and ½ teaspoon

Water – 1 cup

1 teaspoon of honey

<u>INSTRUCTIONS</u>

Step 1

Take a cup of water in a stainless steel bowl or glass bowl and heat it. Remember, green tea turns bitter when it is overheated, so just keep a check on the temperature. Use a kitchen thermometer to see if it's around 85°C.

Step 2

Turn the heat off once it reaches the boiling point. Now, let it cool for a few seconds.

Step 3

Add the green tea powder to the water. The ideal green tea brew time to soak is about 3 minutes, but you may take a sip after 1 ½ minutes to check if the flavor is strong enough.

Step 4

After 3 minutes, the color should have changed to brown. Pour it through a strainer.

Step 5

Add honey to the tea and pour into the cup.

So, this was all about the preparation of green tea in three simple methods. Though this may seem to be easy, the secret of making a perfect cup of green tea lies in the way you brew it. So, here are a few green tea brewing tips that will help you get the right taste and flavor.